Humanizing Prostate Cancer

DI059606

Humanizing Prostate Cancer

A Physician—Patient Perspective

Roger E. Schultz, M.D.
Physician

Alex W. Oliver
Patient

BRANDYLANE PUBLISHERS, INC.

White Stone, Virginia

❋ Brandylane Publishers, Inc.

P.O. Box 261, White Stone, Virginia 22578

(804) 435-6900 or 1 800 553-6922; e-mail: brandy@crosslink.net

Library of Congress Catalog Card Number: 99–40668

Contents

Introduction

This manual is for the thousands of men who have been diagnosed with prostate cancer. Available literature about prostate cancer is often too technical and impersonal. The authors wanted to write a different kind of book to help humanize this frightening experience—a manual that is conversational in tone, easy to read, and sensitive. Their purpose is to convey important information that allows the patient to understand the disease and what can be done about it. They also wanted to talk about the mental and emotional adjustments a man must make once he's been diagnosed, because this is a vital part of healing.

This manual is more than a medical journal filled with the latest research abstracts. What makes this resource different is that it presents a dual perspective—from both a cancer survivor and the urologist who helped him. The patient, Alex Oliver's, comments provide the emotional response many men feel when faced with the diagnosis, but are often unwilling to share openly. His urologist, Roger Schultz, offers plenty of medical data and his experiences in dealing with men faced with this diagnosis. Together, they present a balanced and insightful look at a disease that has become one of the most prevalent among men.

At the least, according to the authors, this is an effort to help men, their families and friends better understand the disease and its treatment. At best, it will help calm frayed nerves and empower men to make intelligent choices about treatment and help them live full lives after treatment.

Acknowledgments

Production Assistance: Betsy Parsons, Helen Potter, Dave Doody, Karen Babb, Susan Bruno, Kem Putney, Jean and Terry Zahn, WHRV-FM-Hear/Say, the American Cancer Society.

Medical Assistance: Milton D. Chalkley, M.D.; Maurice O. Murphy, M.D.; Paul F. Schellhammer, M.D.; Donald F. Lynch, Jr., M.D.; C. Ronald Kersh, M.D.; Patricia Ondercin Ph.D., LCP; Charles Parker, D.O.; Anthony J. Taylor, M.D.; and Judith Korsnick, M.A.

The information in this manual comes from our personal experience and training. It is a guide, but it is not a substitute for the medical opinion that you receive from your own health care provider.

The material in this text is certain to change. There are new developments in medical technology and pharmacology that will alter the way we diagnose and treat prostate cancer in the future.

Chapter 1

Welcome to the Fraternity

You may be among the 185,000 men in the U.S.[1] who have been diagnosed this year with prostate cancer. This is the most common cancer in men over fifty. It is not necessarily fatal. If found early, it can be treated and cured. Even when found in an advanced stage, prostate cancer can be palliated, or slowed down, with hormonal therapy. *There is something that can be done for every man who first presents with newly diagnosed prostate cancer.*

Schultz

Alex was referred to me with an elevated PSA (*prostate specific antigen*) blood test. This blood test has been used both to screen and follow the progress of men with prostate cancer. Alex had no symptoms and his prostate exam felt normal. We did a prostatic biopsy because of the blood test abnormality. Alex will tell you how he reacted.

Oliver

Sweat poured from my brow the moment he said, "You have prostate cancer." With little

[1] "Cancer Facts and Figures," American Cancer Society, 1998.

warning, this physician and this disease captivated my life. I was devastated. Why me? Why now?

Schultz

I've been giving men this news for fifteen years. There's no easy way to say it. Like most men, Alex was pretty shocked. It took time for him to get beyond the words, "prostate cancer," and to absorb any more information. Medical school teaches doctors a new language. Alex has retrained me to put this language back into common English. Most importantly he has also reminded me of the importance of humanizing the entire experience.

Oliver

Immediately my life was different. I became a recluse and my imagination went wild. For the moment, core values, logical thinking and my support group were not within reach. I was terrified.

Schultz

What Alex felt is really no different from any person who learns that he has cancer. Frankly, he was more open about his fear. Most men that I have treated initially clam up and pretend to be strong. Sometimes I meet men who insist that they don't want anyone in their family to know! These fellows would do so much better to involve their most reliable support group—their family or closest friends.

_____ *Oliver*

I was so terrified, I was unsure that I could handle the situation. But I had been taught early on that it was a sign of strength to ask for help. Roger also recognized that counseling would help. Expressing my true emotions to him and letting him be part of the solution helped in making this new stranger become a trusted doctor.

Counseling pinpointed the emotional issue immediately. My fright was due to unresolved memories of my father's illness with cancer. I was six years old when he died. All I remember was his long suffering. During the 1950s, doctors didn't know much about early diagnosis and treatment. There wasn't much anyone could do, and doctors were reluctant to see him at home. Once I realized that considerable progress had been made and that his case was entirely different from mine, I began to calm down. At first, being told I had cancer meant that I was going to die. I'm glad I got help. Soon I began to think more clearly about the emotional side of the disease.

Schultz

With time Alex became better informed about his particular case. We began to talk about the options for treatment. I recall that he would bring a list of questions at every visit. It became obvious that understanding his case helped to reduce his anxiety. In my opinion, it is vital that every man recognize that this is a common condition, that it is treatable when caught early, and that there is a fraternity of men who have been through this process and still maintain normal lives.

Oliver

Occasionally I would call Roger between office visits to ask some questions over again or to make sure I was understanding what he had told me. He always called me back promptly and never seemed bothered with my "what ifs."

> "We can do so many incredible things in medicine, but we often are far too focused on the technical issues of diagnosis and treatment. We should recognize the importance of helping patients cope, educating our patients, and involving family members."
>
> *Roger E. Schultz, M.D.*

> ➤ "The tendency to escalate a situation into its worst possible conclusion is called *awfulizing*, and it can be a key factor in tipping the balance toward illness or health." (Joan Borysenko in *Minding the Body/ Mending the Mind*)

> ➤ Remember, "Make the mind command the body . . . Fear kills more people than death," General Patton.

Schultz

Fear and panic are not constructive emotions. You get better results when you keep your head on straight.

Oliver

In the ensuing weeks that led to surgery, I delved deeply into the physical, mental and emotional aspects of the disease. Soon I became comfortable with what I had to do and confident in my *urologist*. By surgery day, I was ready. In fact, the surgery went beautifully and very much as he had described to me.

> "Generally, bad news makes the best headlines,"
> says Chris Matthews in *Hardball.* The good news is
> that thousands of men who have been diagnosed
> with the disease are living normal lives.
>
> *Alex W. Oliver*

Schultz

We chose surgery for Alex based on his young age, excellent health and clinical circumstances. I believe that Alex did well because he was very prepared and very comfortable with his decision. He was soon back to a normal routine as I had anticipated.

Oliver

In the time since my surgery, I have spoken with numerous men who have been diagnosed with prostate cancer. While each individual has different concerns, there is one similar response —fear!

Schultz

We are convinced that the fear factor can be minimized by the patient and doctor forming a good working relationship. In the best of circumstances, the physician is unhurried and empathetic. It may take several visits to develop a comfort level that permits truly meaningful communication. If the physician can provide his patient with information about the therapy and its risks, the patient will be better prepared to deal with any potential problems or unforeseen circumstances. Also, if a patient is armed with information about the potential risks of therapy, he will be better prepared to deal with any problems that arise following therapy.

Oliver

The relationship with your doctor can be established by being yourself. I liked knowing that he always had good eye contact with me. I was a real person and not just one more name in his patient charts.

> O.K. So now you know you have prostate cancer. At least you know. Just think of the number of men who have it and don't yet know.

> Try not to compare your case, treatment, and/or recovery with anyone else. Each man's story is different.

Alex W. Oliver

Chapter 2

Don't Believe Everything You Hear

Schultz

Alex was troubled by all the hearsay about prostate cancer. Like other men, he couldn't get a handle on what was fact and what was fiction.

Oliver

Once I began to sort the facts and understand my specific case, I began to relax. Contrary to the myth, considerable progress has been made in the detection and treatment of prostate cancer. Many of us who have joined the fraternity are now able to benefit from the more recent research and developments in treatment.

Schultz

First, let's begin by identifying the location of the prostate.

Where is the prostate located?

The prostate sits beneath the bladder and surrounds the urethra.

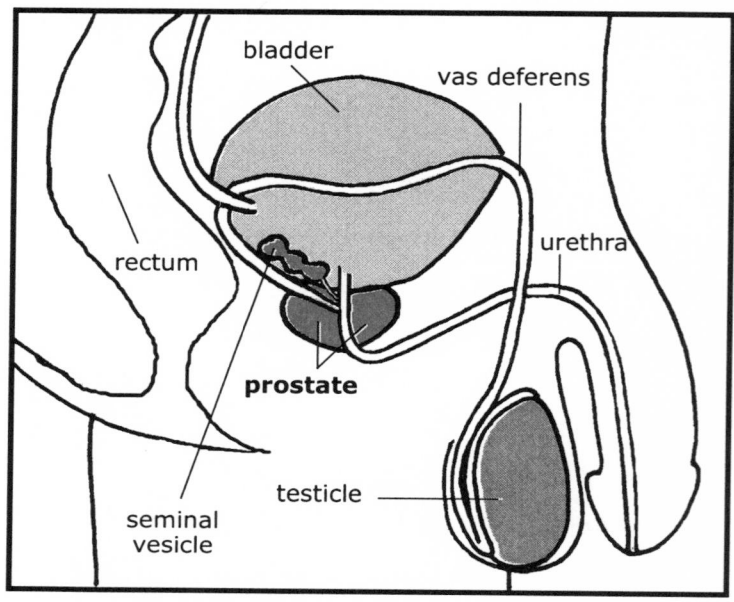

We feel that it is important to point out some of the ideas about this disease that are false.

Exploring the Myths and Realities

The prostate's job is to help with sex.

After puberty, the prostate makes semen. After age fifty, it makes trouble! It is the most common organ to develop cancer in men over fifty. The prostate has nothing to do with sex drive, erections, and orgasm. The nerves and blood vessels that go to the penis pass on either side of the prostate. An injury to these structures, but not the prostate itself, can lead to problems with erections.

There must be something in the air or water. More men are getting the disease.

We are finding more cases of prostate cancer because of the PSA (Prostate Specific Antigen) test and a greater awareness about the disease. Fatty foods may be related, but not the air or water. You are at greater risk of developing prostate cancer if you are older, African-American, or have a father or brother with the same disease.

This is an old man's disease, so I can ignore it until I retire.

Not true! With the arrival of the PSA blood test, doctors have identified men in their fifties and sixties who have normal prostate examinations and no symptoms. The biopsies of their prostates often show higher grades of cancer, sometimes lots of it too.

Get a PSA test, but forget the rectal exam!

These tests complement one another, so both should be done. About 25% of men with prostate cancer have a normal PSA. The cancer may show up as a nodule (hard spot) felt by examination. So don't talk your doctor out of the *digital rectal exam.*

Prostate cancer is slow growing and you'll outlive it, so why bother looking for it.

This might be true for a very old man with a tiny area of prostate cancer found on a biopsy. On the other hand, it might be risky for a healthy fifty year old to ignore his diagnosis and take the chance that the tumor will never affect him. Why? Because the cancer inevitably grows. Once the cancer spreads, there is no treatment that will cure or eliminate the cancer. Advanced disease can be painful and costly. In later chapters we will review how the *grade* and the *volume* of cancer affect prognosis.

Life is never the same after treatment. Your sex life ends and you leak urine constantly.

If we treat a man whose cancer is confined to the prostate, he will likely return to a normal working life. Treatment for advanced stages will generally control the tumor and either improve or delay the appearance of symptoms such as bone pain, urinary bleeding or urinary obstruction.

Impotence (inability to get good erections) may occur with treatment. The newer techniques (e.g., nerve sparing surgery, conformal radiation, and brachytherapy) can lessen the likelihood of impotence. There are many different ways to treat men with erectile dysfunction, so don't write off your sex life!

Urinary incontinence (leakage) rarely occurs with radiation, but might occur after surgery. Some men will have stress incontinence—leakage that occurs with coughing or swinging a golf club. This often improves with time, and it can be treated if it persists. Your age, body build, and general health influence this potential problem, so you should discuss this issue with your urologist.

I have to have my treatment at a cancer institute.

If your Ford breaks down, do you take it to Detroit for repairs? Having a choice of treatments is better than no choice at all, but it does create confusion and anxiety. I often advise patients to seek a second or third opinion from other doctors, including those at major medical centers. Once you decide on treatment, then you must choose the treating doctor. This depends on your confidence in your physician. Does he have credentials? Is he well regarded by his medical peers? Does he take time to explain? Does he listen to you? A busy community *urologist* or *radiation oncologist* may provide care that is as good as the cancer centers. You will need someone to call if you have any problems related to your treatment. And you will need follow-up to be sure that you remain free of cancer. This is a lot more easily done if you develop a relationship with a doctor near your home and hospital.

We haven't made much progress in the diagnosis or treatment of this disease.

Not so! I can show you major developments in both diagnosis and treatment.

In the area of diagnosis, the PSA blood test has allowed earlier detection. Ultrasound allows us to see deep inside the prostate gland.

Biopsy instruments are smaller, faster, and less painful.

In the treatment arena, surgery is more routine than ever. Because of newer techniques, complications, particularly urinary incontinence and impotence, are much less common. Conformal *external beam irradiation* allows the treating doctor to wrap the radiation around the prostate, minimizing risk to the nearby organs like the bladder and rectum. *Brachytherapy*, the placement of radioactive seeds in the prostate, is gaining popularity due to improved imaging that allows more accurate distribution of seeds.

The use of newer hormonal shots and oral drugs called *antiandrogens* have allowed excellent *palliation* of advanced disease. Newer chemotherapy drugs have shown improved response rates even in cases that would not respond to other treatments.

Genetic research is the hot subject today. We may soon be able to analyze genes and predict whether a man is at risk for prostate cancer. There is hope that we may one day insert or remove genes in our DNA that will protect us from cancer and/or inhibit the growth of cancer cells.

Chapter 3

A New Chapter in Your Life

Oliver

Please note that we call this "A New Chapter In Your Life" not "The Last Word." What we offer in this chapter are basic facts, many of which may be new to you. Understanding the diagnosis will help you to determine the course of treatment. We believe having a basic understanding will also help quiet the alarm bell.

Understanding the Diagnosis

Schultz

A tumor is a growth that occurs in a body organ that may or may not be life threatening. Speaking very generally, a benign tumor usually remains confined to the same organ from which it began. A malignant tumor is one that can grow out of control and spread to other organs. A malignant tumor is called a cancer. When cancer spreads to other organs, it can interfere with the function of those organs. It can weaken the body's immune system, that is, the ability to fight off even simple infections. The cancer saps the nutrition from healthy cells and can cause weight loss and weakness. People die from cancer for many reasons, but the most common ones are severe infections and the failure of multiple organs.

Remember that early prostate cancer may cause no symptoms. We have already discussed the importance of an annual *digital rectal examination* and *PSA blood test* for those men who wish to screen for prostate cancer. The PSA blood test can be falsely elevated by benign prostatic enlargement or prostatitis (inflammation). Passing instruments or catheters into the bladder may elevate it. It is not elevated by simple rectal examination of the prostate. If there is any question regarding the validity of the PSA result, I would repeat it. If there are signs or symptoms of prostatitis (genital pain, soft/tender prostate to examination), I will treat it and then repeat the PSA in six weeks to see if there is a significant decrease in value. If the digital rectal examination or the PSA is abnormal, we would advise a prostate biopsy under ultrasound guidance. This is an office-based test that takes just fifteen minutes. We pass an ultrasound probe about two inches in the rectum and use it to guide a biopsy device to several areas of the prostate. The instrument has a small needle that fires quickly. There is some discomfort, often a desire to urinate, but rarely significant pain. I do not feel sedation is necessary. Multiple biopsies are taken to see if cancer is present and to estimate its extent in the prostate (volume of disease).

Oliver

For me there was no pain resulting from the test. I was tired but that was caused by my anxiety.

> ➤ You don't have to play Tarzan when going through therapy. Let your body tell you what you can do. Learn to relax and work on total self-healing.
> *Alex W. Oliver*

> ➤ Part of the fraternity initiation is experiencing "data shock" (*So much new information to understand so quickly*). Let your physician help you through the crisis. He is on your side and is your best resource. Ask questions.
>
> *Alex W. Oliver*

Schultz

Cancer is usually diagnosed by a *pathologist*, a physician skilled at recognizing cancer when the specimens are viewed under a microscope. He will assign a *grade* to the cancer. This is an attempt to judge how aggressive the cancer may behave. The grade is based on the appearance of the cells and their relationship to other cells.

One of the most popular grading systems was described by *Gleason*. He defines five microscopic patterns of prostate cancer and gives each pattern a number from one (least aggressive) to five (most aggressive). He then adds the two most common patterns seen under the microscope, giving him the *Gleason score*. A low Gleason score (e.g., 3+2=5) generally has a better prognosis than a high Gleason score (e.g., 4+5=9). Like pieces of a puzzle, the combination of PSA level, Gleason score, and tumor volume tell us about tumor behavior.

Staging the Disease

We discover prostate cancer at different stages. The *stage* refers to the location of the cancer relative to the rest of the body. Is the cancer well within the borders of the prostate? Has it broken through the prostate capsule into the fatty tissue around the prostate? Has it spread to other organs (e.g., the bones or the lungs)?

There are two staging systems that are popular among physicians. The first is the *Whitmore-Jewett system* of four stages (A, B, C & D). The other is the *TNM system* which is more universally known and shown in Table 1. The "T" refers to Tumor size. The "N" refers to the lymph node status. The "M" refers to the presence of metastases (cancer spread).

Using the TNM system, we categorize a man with cancer found only by way of elevated PSA as a stage T1. If there is a nodule, it is a T2. A larger cancer has a higher T number. With regard to spread to lymph nodes and other organs, we will often order a CAT scan of the pelvis, a bone scan, a chest X-ray, and blood tests that check your blood count or liver function. Recent clinical research has shown that many of these tests are not needed if the Gleason score is less than 6 and the PSA is less than 10 ng/ml. In this instance, the likelihood of finding cancer beyond the prostate is so low that these tests may be a waste of time and money. A newer nuclear scan, called Prostascint, has also been developed to look for the spread of prostate cancer. It has not been universally accepted for staging because the results may not be reliable.

TABLE 1: TNM System for Staging Prostate Cancer

T ➤ **Primary Tumor**

  TX ➤ Primary tumor cannot be assessed.

  T1 ➤ Cannot feel tumor or see it using imaging (x-ray or ultrasound). Cancer found in specimen after a transurethral resection of prostate. Cancer found on a biopsy done only because of an elevated PSA test.

  T2 ➤ Tumor is confined to the prostate.

  T3 ➤ Tumor breaks through the capsule of the prostate or invades the seminal vesicles.

  T4 ➤ Tumor invades structures other than the seminal vesicles.

N ➤ **Regional Lymph Nodes**

  NX ➤ Regional lymph nodes cannot be assessed.

  N0 ➤ Regional lymph nodes do not show cancer present.

  N1 ➤ Regional lymph nodes contain cancer.

M ➤ **Distant metastasis (cancer spread)**

  MX ➤ Distant metastases cannot be assessed.

  M0 ➤ No distant metastases seen.

  M1 ➤ Distant metastases are present.

There is yet another blood test called *PCR* which might detect microscopic amounts of circulating PSA in the blood. Sounds like it's useful, but the methodology and results with PCR vary from site to site. It has not been endorsed for staging by most urologists. Much like the chapter on therapy, you can find a multitude of tests that could be done, but someone educated in the treatment of this disease needs to help you choose those tests that assist decision-making and minimize anxiety.

Chapter 4

Choices and Challenges

Oliver

My first reaction to the diagnosis was to do something quickly. In most cases you will have time to determine what is best for you. Don't panic. Get the facts. There may be several treatment options. I had three choices. My wife and I agreed that surgery was my best option. The doctor agreed. The three of us were partners in making the medical decision.

My friends tell me I was totally absorbed in this crisis and they didn't know how to help. I didn't know any man who had survived prostate cancer. More discussion would have helped.

Schultz

How do you pick a plan for the treatment of prostate cancer? In the medical community you could speak to your family doctor, urologist, or radiation oncologist. You could do research in the medical library, only to be frustrated by medical technotalk. Others surf the Net and find reams of data. Or you could contact sources who provide integrative medicine. Unfortunately, there are very few clinical trials that prove that alternative approaches alone will cure prostate cancer. On the other hand, there is data to suggest that proper exercise, nutrition, and stress reduction will strengthen the body and boost its immune system.

First and foremost, I suggest that you find a physician whom you trust and who is an expert in this disease. Seek additional opinion if you feel so inclined. Talk to friends or survivors within support groups (like Us Too; Man to Man. See below), but recognize that their circumstances are not always comparable to your own. Get your loved ones involved. If you are supported, if you collect information that can be sorted and interpreted, if you trust your advisors, then you will be able to take charge, make a decision, and promote your own healing.

Prostate Cancer Support Groups
Call to find out local chapter information.

Man to Man
Supported by the American Cancer Society
1-800-ACS-2345

Us Too International
1-800-808-7866

> ➤ There is no best approach for all cancers. The first thing I tell patients is that they have to decide whether they will treat the disease or not. If they choose treatment, then they can select from a menu of options. The decision to treat will depend upon multiple issues: the age and general mental, emotional and physical health of the patient, the grade/stage of disease, the PSA level, and the expectations and fears of the individual.
>
> *Roger E. Schultz, M.D.*

Let's explore each option and look at some examples.

Watchful Waiting

Schultz

I never did like this term. It sounds as if we are waiting for disaster to occur. I prefer 'observation only.' The tumor is very small. The pathologist has given it a low Gleason score. Your PSA may be normal or only minimally elevated. In this case, we would keep an eye on the PSA and clinical signs and symptoms. Should there be a dramatic change in either, we could start treatment.

Example: A seventy-two year old man has a *transurethral resection of the prostate* (*TURP*, "ream-job") to help him urinate more easily. Although his PSA and prostate exam are normal, the tissue removed shows a tiny spot of cancer in less than 1% of the specimen (Gleason score = 3). He chooses no treatment. Over time there is no change in the PSA or prostate exam. He continues to urinate easily and has no problems related to his prostate.

> The benefit of observation only is clearly the lack of any of the side effects or the expense of treatment. The disadvantage is the remote possibility of cancer spreading to other areas of the body.
>
> *Roger E. Schultz*

External Beam Irradiation

Schultz

If the prostate tumor is T3 or less and there is no spread of disease, you may benefit from this form of therapy. Recent information suggests that the use of hormonal shots given in and around the time of the radiation may shrink the prostate and improve the response to the radiation. You would be asked to go to a radiation oncologist for consultation. They would decide the proper dosing of radiation. You would be scheduled to come back daily for a brief exposure to radiation aimed at the prostate. The newest technique of conformal therapy allows them to wrap the radiation around the prostate in a way that minimizes radiation scatter to the nearby bladder or rectum. The radiation must be given in small amounts over about an eight week period. It destroys the tumor while leaving the prostate in place. The results are judged by the prostate exam (it often feels flat after treatment) and the PSA level. The PSA "nadir" (the lowest level to which the PSA should decrease) is debatable. Some say it should fall to less than 4 ng/ml if the cancer has been destroyed. Others feel it should fall to less than 0.5 ng/ml. Regardless of the absolute value, all agree that the PSA should not rise from its lower baseline over several consecutive visits. A PSA that rises off its new baseline suggests that the cancer is still active.

Example: A seventy-two year old man has a hard area involving the entire right side of the prostate. The PSA is 8ng/ml. Biopsy confirms a cancer with a Gleason score = 6. He has coronary artery disease and diabetes that is controlled with insulin.

In this example, surgery may not be ideal. First of all, his heart disease and diabetes increase the risk of surgical complications (heart attack, infection). Second, if the tumor is large and may extend beyond the confines of the prostate, he may need additional therapy, possibly radiation! So it may be wiser to direct this man to radiation first.

Brachytherapy

Schultz

Brachytherapy or interstitial irradiation is the placement of radioactive "seeds" directly in the prostate gland. The seeds emit radiation that kills prostate cancer cells, then they "burn out." Over time the seeds lose their radioactivity and remain in the prostate gland forever. In the past, brachytherapy was not as successful as other treatments because of the limitations of the technique to insert them. We had to make an abdominal incision and push needles into the prostate through which the seeds were passed. Much of the procedure was done by feel, so it was not surprising that there was often an uneven distribution of seeds. Our failure to reliably control the disease may have been due to recurrent cancer in areas of the prostate that were never irradiated.

During the past several years there has been renewed interest in brachytherapy because of improved techniques to map the prostate using computers and because of improved delivery systems using ultrasound. Brachytherapy is a cooperative effort between the urologist and the radiation oncologist. We first measure the prostate volume by placing an ultrasound probe in the rectum. Multiple images are taken and a computer helps to determine the total volume. These measurements help us decide how many seeds may be needed to treat the entire gland. We order the seeds and schedule the treatment itself. On the day of treatment you are taken to the operating room, given an anesthetic and placed in stirrups. A grid is placed up against the perineum (area between the scrotal sac and the rectum). We put the ultrasound probe in the rectum to identify the prostate and guide the process. Needles are placed through the holes in the grid and seeds are then passed down the center of these needles into the prostate gland. We remove the needles leaving the seeds behind. You go home the same day. Some doctors combine external beam irradiation and brachytherapy for higher grade (more aggressive) cancer.

Example: A sixty-seven year old healthy man has a small prostate with a nodule. Biopsy confirms a Gleason score = 5 in the nodule only. This patient wants to be cured, and he wants a minimally invasive approach to therapy. Although he could choose external beam radiation or surgery, he opts instead for brachytherapy. He accepts the fact that, at this time, we have less data available on the long term cure rates using this approach.

Surgery

Schultz

The surgical removal of prostate cancer is called a *radical prostatectomy*. The term *radical* refers to the complete removal of the entire prostate and *seminal vesicles*. People ask why we can't remove the cancerous area and leave the normal prostate gland alone. This is because prostate cancer is often found or may develop in multiple areas within the gland. It is also technically harder to cut out a segment of this single, centrally placed organ.

The nerves that go to the penis to provide an erection sit alongside the prostate. When possible, the surgeon will try to protect these nerves as he removes the prostate. When the prostate has been removed, the surgeon must sew the bladder to the urethral stump. A urethral catheter (Foley) is left in place for several weeks until the connection between the bladder and urethra has a watertight seal. The operation takes about two to four hours. The hospital stay is about two to four days.

There is some debate whether hormone treatments should be given prior to surgery in an effort to shrink the gland and increase the likelihood of removal of all the cancer. At this time, the use of pre-operative hormonal treatment is not the standard of care.

Why would you choose surgery instead of radiation? Surgery is faster (two to four hours vs. eight weeks for external beam irradiation). Surgery is the only way to actually hand examine and learn more about the patient's prognosis. Some argue that surgery provides a better cure rate, particularly if the tumor appears aggressive (high Gleason score). Nerve sparing surgery may permit a greater likelihood of erections after treatment. Finally, if cancer shows up again in the pelvis, you can undergo radiation to this area. The reverse is not as easy. If you have recurrent cancer after radiation treatment, it is not possible to undergo more pelvic irradiation, and surgery on tissues that have received radiation is very difficult.

Example: A fifty year old athletic man is sent to us following annual physical because his PSA = 5.0 ng/ml. He has no symptoms and his prostate feels normal. Biopsy confirms a Gleason score 5 prostate cancer in two of six cores sent. He is potent and wants to remain so! He would have a high likelihood of cure with few complications if he chose surgery.

Cryoablative Surgery

Schultz

This procedure involves the placement of a probe in the rectum which is used to freeze and destroy the tumor. Some doctors and patients feel that this procedure has been prematurely dismissed as ineffective. There is concern that *cryosurgery* does not fully destroy all the cancer. Sometimes there can be serious injury to the rectum. I usually present this option to patients; however, it is among the least utilized primary treatments.

Hormonal deprivation

Schultz

Prostate cancer is sensitive to the effects of testosterone, a hormone produced mostly by the testicles and a little by the adrenal glands. We can slow down the activity of prostate cancer by removing the testicles (*orchiectomies*). This is done as an outpatient and takes about thirty minutes.

Drug therapy is an alternative to removal of the testicles. In the past we offered a pill called Diethylstilbestrol (DES). This medication had some undesirable side effects (breast enlargement, hypercoagulability of blood which could cause a stroke). We now offer newer medication called *LHRH agonists* (e.g., Lupron, Zoladex). These are shots that can last from one to four months depending on the preparation. They must be given continually. The medication is no more effective than surgery. It is only an alternative, and a costly alternative, at that! All of these treatments will cause hot flashes and impotence.

Some, but not all doctors believe that the small amount of testosterone generated by the adrenal gland should also be eliminated to maximize survival. This can be done using oral drugs called *antiandrogens* (Eulexin, Casodex, Nilandron). These medicines may be given whether you choose orchiectomies or LHRH shots. The combination is referred to as *complete androgen blockade*. Given the high costs of these medicines, you should discuss this issue with your doctor.

Hormonal deprivation is not typically offered to a man with a potentially curable cancer. Although the cancer may shrink away initially, it will eventually become resistant to the effects of orchiectomies or LHRH shots. Unresponsive cells start to grow and can cause urinary symptoms or spread farther.

Example: A fifty-five year old man has some trouble voiding. His prostate is not large, but it is uniformly rock hard. His PSA is 45 ng/ml! Biopsy confirms a Gleason score 9 cancer in six of six cores sent. A bone scan shows "hot spots" (*metastases*) in numerous areas in his ribs and pelvic bones.

Neither prostatectomy nor radiation of any kind will cure him. Hormonal deprivation gives a high likelihood of controlling the growth of his cancer for several months or possibly several years. A recurrence is very likely.

Schultz

Chemotherapy is not a primary treatment for most prostate cancers. It is generally reserved for cases in which hormonal deprivation has failed. Chemotherapy may slow tumor growth and may relieve pain. Some of the drugs used alone, or in combination, include Prednisone, Mitoxantrone, Estramustine, Doxorubicin, Etoposide, Vinblastine, and Paclitaxel. The prognosis with cancer that does not respond to chemotherapy is poor.

Oliver

In my case, the doctor suggested several choices for therapy: surgery, radiation, or brachytherapy. What is most important is that we made the final decision for surgery together.

Chapter 5

We Thought You'd Never Ask!

If you don't learn anything else from our manual, please remember to ask your doctor as many questions as you need answers. We've even done some thinking for you by giving you eighteen questions and answers. If there are others, write them down and ask them during your next visit.

Schultz

Your doctor sees a great number of patients on a regular basis. Don't expect him to anticipate all of your questions. It is up to you to get the facts you need in making the best decision. Remember, the only dumb questions are the ones you didn't ask!

Eighteen Questions for Your Physician

1. What is the normal range for the PSA (prostate specific antigen) blood test?

The value for PSA increases with age. There are several different methods of measuring PSA, so you must ask your doctor about his lab's reference ranges. For example, using the

Hybritech method of measuring PSA, the range can be from 2.5-6.5 ng/ml depending upon the age. A PSA = 4.0 may be abnormally high for a forty year old, but well within the normal range for a seventy year old. The rate of change of PSA from test to test is also important. A rapidly rising PSA between doctor visits can also indicate a possible cancer. If your PSA is borderline and/ or slowly rising, we may order a *Percent Free-PSA* blood test. This measures how much PSA is free versus how much is bound to other blood proteins. If your Percent Free–PSA is *low* (low is abnormal), you may need a prostate biopsy.

2. How do I know whether my doctor is qualified to advise or treat me?

You should certainly lean on your family physician for initial guidance. He will likely steer you to a urologist, a radiation oncologist, or both. Look for Board Certification, a qualification that tells you that the doctor has passed some difficult exams given by his peers. Ask what his/her experience has been treating prostate cancer. Ask if there is a similar patient in his practice who would be willing to speak to you about his experience.

➢ Don't expect your doctor to speak in absolute terms. "Always" and "never" are not in his vocabulary.

Alex W. Oliver

3. Who else could I contact for information?

There are Prostate Cancer Support groups (Us Too, Man to Man and others) in most areas with larger populations. Some other suggestions include the Prostate Cancer Network of the American Foundation for Urologic Diseases (800-828-7866), the Prostate Information Center (800-543-9632), the National Cancer Institute (800-4-CANCER) and the American Cancer Society (404-320-3333).

4. How quickly must I act?

This depends on your PSA level, your biopsy report, your health, and your anxiety level. In cases of early detection, there is very limited risk in waiting several weeks to gather information. You should be able to get it all together within a few weeks. More advanced cases may need more urgent treatment.

5. What happens if I don't do anything?

Again, this depends on the status of your disease (PSA level, Gleason score, cancer volume). If you have early disease and no symptoms, you might not have any problems for months or even years. In most instances, prostate cancer grows slowly, but it invariably grows! Once the disease is more advanced, it can cause a variety of symptoms: urinary (weak stream, urgent need to void, bloody urine), bone pain, obstructed kidneys, weight loss, and weakness.

6. How much should I tell my family, friends, and co-workers?

In our opinion, you should involve your closest family members or friends in the decision process. Who else cares more for you? There is no shame in telling your friends or work mates who ask about your condition. You may prompt them to get a check-up also!

7. Can I hurt myself or my partner by having sex?

Prostate cancer is not contagious! Sexual intimacy of any kind will not make your cancer worse, nor will it cause any harm to your partner.

8. Does insurance pay for the tests and the treatment for prostate cancer?

Your medical insurance will pay unless your doctor orders unusual or uncommon tests or treatments. If you are concerned, call your insurance carrier before you proceed.

9. Doesn't radical prostatectomy cause incontinence and impotence?

You need a seasoned surgeon to get good results. Continual urinary leakage should be very rare. Some men will have stress incontinence, a little drip when they are physically active. Obese men have a greater risk of urinary leakage after surgery.

The nerve sparing prostatectomy really does work. Erectile function can take up to a year or more to fully return. Best results are in younger, very potent men. Men over the age of seventy may not retain the quality of erections they had earlier.

10. What is the difference between a radical perineal prostatectomy and a radical retropubic prostatectomy?

The perineal approach involves an incision just above the anus. Generally, the perineal approach is less bloody and allows the patient to go home about one day sooner than the abdominal approach. So why don't all urologists do the perineal prostatectomy? There are several reasons, not the least of which is the training and experience of the surgeon. Both procedures get the job done, but some urology training programs emphasize the perineal and others like the retropubic approach.

The retropubic surgery is done through a lower abdominal incision. There are two advantages. First, we can sample the lymph nodes near the prostate. If the nodes have cancer, we may stop the operation and close because we will be unlikely to cure the patient by removing the prostate. Nerve sparing surgery may also be more effective with a retropubic approach.

11. *What are the side effects of radiation?*

The bladder and rectum can be affected by radiation "scatter." This translates into urinary urgency/frequency and rectal discomfort/diarrhea. These symptoms can be treated and they usually disappear once the radiation treatment has been completed. Some men develop troublesome, long term rectal or bladder bleeding.

12. *Why doesn't everyone select brachytherapy if it can be done as an outpatient?*

If you wish to avoid or cannot undergo surgery, this is a viable alternative. This procedure cannot be done if the prostate is very large because we will be unable to treat the entire gland, especially that portion that projects behind the pubic bone. Patients who have had previous prostate surgery are also poor candidates for brachytherapy. There is growing interest in this procedure, but it does not yet have the long track record of surgery or external beam irradiation. Many doctors are concerned that the distribution of seeds may be uneven and may not destroy the entire tumor. Brachytherapy is not available in all areas because of lack of equipment and training in this technique.

---

13. What do I do if surgery fails to control the cancer? If radiation fails?

If there is a late recurrence of cancer after surgery, and if we feel that this is due to a pelvic recurrence (at the surgical site), then you can undergo external beam irradiation to the pelvis. If the recurrence is distant (*metastatic*), you will need hormonal treatment.

If there is a pelvic recurrence after radiation of any kind, you have a bigger problem. You cannot receive additional radiation. "Salvage prostatectomy" can be done, but the surgery of irradiated tissue is difficult. Complications of impotence and incontinence are much higher after salvage surgery. Cryotherapy is an option, but there is not much data to wholeheartedly advise it. Hormonal treatment is often advised as *palliation*.

14. Which is better for palliation of advanced disease— removal of testicles (orchiectomies) or shots (LHRH agonists)?

Neither is better. Both accomplish the same thing by lowering serum testosterone. There is no benefit to doing both orchiectomies and shots. The choice is strictly a personal one. Removal of the testicles takes thirty minutes in the operating room. It is a one time treatment, and it is permanent. The LHRH shots wear off and must be given repeatedly. The shots are very expensive but generally covered by insurance.

15. What is pulse or intermittent therapy using LHRH shots?

We give the LHRH shots on a fixed schedule, every three to four months depending on the product used. Some doctors are exploring the use of administering the drug only if and when there are changes in the PSA, exam, or symptoms. This would lessen the cost and side effects of these drugs. This is not common practice at this time.

16. What can I do to prevent prostate cancer?

Stay on a diet that is low in animal fat. I support patients who wish to take Vitamin E, antioxidants, selenium, or green tea, but in all honesty, I have not seen data that shows a proven benefit in a large series of men who use these products. Studies are underway to see whether Finasteride (Proscar) can prevent this disease.

17. If I have had prostatitis, am I at increased risk for prostate cancer?

Not to my knowledge.

18. I get mailings about drugs that improve prostate health. Most of these drugs are non-prescription. Do they work?

In my opinion, the unsolicited mailings are simply ads. Most doctors have been taught to use medication that has clear benefits when compared to a placebo (a blank pill containing no medicine). There is little or no data to suggest that a non-prescriptive drug will cure prostate cancer any better than a placebo.

Chapter 6

Getting It Together

Schultz

The medical profession has made significant advances in the treatment of prostate cancer. One of the most important findings is that men who are prepared mentally, physically, and spiritually do much better with treatment and recovery. Alex is a good example of a young man who worked through the fright and anger stages and did well with treatment.

Oliver

Take a quick look at the front cover. What does the yellow square with the red dot mean to you? Responses will vary, but there is a 99.5% chance that your answer had something to do with the red dot.

Is there a lesson to this exercise? You bet! Think of the square as your total life. Don't allow the red dot to overshadow the yellow surface.

To be more specific, don't let prostate cancer become your life. Easy to say? Harder to do? Yes! Take it from one whose life became a red square for a while. And, boy, was it unnecessary!

So take a few tips from one who learned the hard way.

Avoid fantasizing about what could happen.

Ask your doctor specific questions that can reduce the fear. Write down the answers. Every time you find yourself slipping into the fear zone, read the "awfulizing" quote on page 5.

Learn what you must let go and what you can control.

This was hard for me, a professional control freak. It didn't take long to find out that the doctor, the quarterback, was in charge of much of my life. What helped me was understanding what I could control: my physical and spiritual well-being; my understanding of the disease and my particular case; my handling of my work and social schedule to meet the requirements of appointments and testing schedule. In short, I could be in control of life up to a point. But it was fine with me for Roger to be my partner in making medical decisions. I had confidence in him.

Although I did not know Roger Schultz, I knew of his reputation in the medical community and from other men he had treated. Roger told me that surgery had been fine-tuned and that I would very likely do well. He was right.

I had surgery on a Thursday morning. By Friday afternoon I was up and doing some walking. I ate well and slept comfortably. By Sunday afternoon I was home. Monday I sat at a card table and did a limited amount of work. I experienced little pain and noted an increase in strength every pday. Two weeks later the catheter was removed. No big deal. No pain.

If you think you want a nice, mannerly urologist to handle your case, you agree with me. But let me take it a step further. Be sure he is board certified and that he has experience with prostate cancer.

Did I get a second opinion? No. Why? My case was not that complicated and I felt confident in his ability.

Schultz

Any responsible doctor will tell you if a second opinion is recommended.

When should you get a second or third opinion?

➤ Any time you are not comfortable with the doctor.

➤ When there is not a clear-cut diagnosis or when you want more information.

➤ When you feel you want a second opinion.

WARNING: You could be in a state of denial if you continue to get numerous opinions.

Communicate, communicate, communicate.

It was difficult and somewhat embarrassing for me to talk about this at first. But talking to others does help. Find at least one person you can be honest with. REMEMBER: Even though it's your prostate, the crisis affects your family, friends, and co-workers. I found that the more I talked about it, the more I helped myself.

Did the doctor know how I felt? You bet, and I had no problem leaning on him. After all, he was not only treating the cancer, he was treating me in other ways.

Schultz: Now let me say one more word here. As a doctor, I have found that a former patient can be a great asset to me. In fact, Alex has spoken with many men since his experience. What he tells them is good, practical medicine:

➤ Get exercise. Stay fit.

➤ Eat sensibly.

➤ Get plenty of rest.

➤ Understand your emotional self. If you feel like you're falling down a well or feel tired and angry, talk it out with someone.

➤ Visit the location for your treatment and know who will be there to help you.

➤ Let your coworkers know what your schedule will be during treatment and how they can help you at work.

➤ Allow friends and neighbors to help you with household chores and other responsibilities. Ask them to keep you in their thoughts and prayers.

This can be a stressful time in your life. Taking care of your total self will help.

I have noted a great change in men's attitudes about prostate cancer. We are talking about it and want to help other men. This aids the healing process.

Chapter 7

Life After Therapy

Schultz

Believe it or not, you can resume a normal life following treatment for prostate cancer. You may have restricted activities following surgery for a total of six weeks. After this time, you can gradually resume just about everything you used to do. The side effects of radiation usually don't last long, so you can expect to feel more normal within several weeks or, more rarely, several months following therapy. Hormonal treatments do not limit your physical activities, but the loss of testosterone (male hormone) can make you feel tired and may cause osteoporosis (loss of calcium from bones).

All of these therapies may have one common side effect—erectile impotence. After surgery or radiation, you may need to wait as long as one or two years to see the return of erectile function. With hormonal therapy, your testosterone levels fall and impotence is permanent. You should not write off your sex life, however, because there are several avenues of treatment for this condition regardless of its cause. Your urologist can show you a vacuum constriction device that mechanically helps you to achieve and hold an erection. There are also pharmacological approaches that use drugs that vasodilate, or open up, the penile blood vessels. The most popular right now is Viagra, an oral pill. Another popular product is MUSE, a medicated suppository that you place about one inch down the urethra. The pellet melts and causes an erection in ten minutes. Last, there is a drug called Prostaglandin E-1 which you can inject directly into the penis which will cause an erection within ten minutes.

Except for hormonal therapy, you can expect to retain your interest in sex. Orgasm and the rhythmic muscular contractions that accompany the climax can still occur. There is no significant semen with climax because the source of this fluid, the prostate and seminal vesicles, have been removed or irradiated. Although this affects your fertility, it does not pose any risk to your health.

When neither the vacuum pump nor drugs prove satisfactory, we can recommend the placement of a penile prosthesis. The surgery takes one or two hours and can be done with a very minimal hospital stay. The prosthesis is permanent, but you are no more aware of it than you are aware of the shoe on your foot. It can be used any time and any number of times. The greatest advantage of a penile prosthesis is the spontaneity that it offers. There is no prescription and no special preparation involved. Medicare and many insurance carriers will cover the surgical costs.

Fortunately, most men regain urinary control after radical prostatectomy. Some men have very troubling urgency following surgery. This may be due to a bladder made irritable by previous prostatic obstruction. In these instances, we may offer you an anticholinergic pill (e.g., Detrol, Ditropan) to decrease symptoms. On occasion men develop more severe incontinence. In these cases we may recommend the surgical implantation of an *Artificial Urinary Sphincter (AUS)*. Much like the penile implant, an AUS is a simple one hour procedure, often done with minimal hospital stay. A urethral cuff is implanted which is continuously filled with water to close off the urethra. When you need to void, you simply press a scrotally placed pump to force fluid from the urethral cuff to the reservoir. The bladder will drain out of the opened urethra. In three minutes, the urethral cuff automatically refills and closes the urethra.

> ➤ "My wife, Libbey, tells me that I was tied up in a big knot when I got the news. It was a great deal to think about and I was mostly concerned as to how this could negatively affect my marriage. Libbey worked with me and with time the knot began to unravel. Today my marriage is stronger because of the experience, and the remaining threads of the knot have been woven deeply in the fabric of our lives."
>
> *Alex W. Oliver*

Schultz

I make a big point about follow-up. There is no such thing as a 100% cure rate. Even when we are dealing with locally confined disease, there will be some unfortunate person whose cancer shows up again, either soon after treatment or even years later. Presumably this is due to cancer cells either in the pelvis or in more distant locations. The PSA is the most sensitive marker of recurrent disease. After radical prostatectomy, the PSA should remain undetectable. After successful radiation, the PSA will reach a low level, preferably less than 1 ng/ml, and remain in this range forever. A rising PSA following any treatment generally means recurrent cancer. Some feel that early and rapid rise in PSA after treatment means *metastatic disease.* A late and slow rise after several years may indicate a recurrence in the pelvis, near the site of treatment.

I see my patients several times in the first year following treatment, then less often as time passes without recurrent cancer. At the very least, I see my patients annually. I ask my patients to obtain a PSA one week before their office visits. Recurrent cancer is usually first suggested by a rising PSA in a patient without complaints. The PSA rise may precede the onset of symptoms by many months. Eventually the patient may show up with problems urinating, blood in the urine, unexplained weight loss, or bone pain. Hopefully we can intervene before bigger problems are evident.

Antiandrogens—Oral drugs (Eulexin, Casodex, Nilandron) that block the effects of testosterone. Often used together with either orchiectomies or LHRH agonists in an effort to improve survival.

Brachytherapy (Interstitial radiation)—The placement of radioactive seeds into the substance of the prostate to destroy cancer cells. The seeds are permanently implanted and become inert after many months.

Complete Androgen Blockade—The combination of orchiectomies and antiandrogens, or LHRH agonists and antiandrogens. This will block the production and/or effects of the testosterone produced by the testicles and adrenal glands. It is used in advanced cancer to produce a *remission*.

Digital Rectal Examination—The placement of a finger in the rectum to feel the prostate for its size and shape. Lumps (nodules) are considered unusual and could be cancer.

External beam irradiation—Treatment of prostate cancer by aiming a linear accelerator at the cancer to destroy it. Treatments are given during brief daily visits over an eight week period.

Gleason Score—A system for determining the prognosis. The pathologist views the cancer under the microscope to determine the two most common grades (see Grade). These numbers are added together to give the Gleason score. This can range from 2 (1+1) to 10 (5+5). Higher Gleason scores suggest a worse prognosis.

Grade—A means of deciding the speed of growth of a cancer by looking at the cancer cells under the microscope. Prostate cancer is graded from 1-5. The higher the grade, the more aggressive the tumor.

Hormonal deprivation—Prostate cancer often shrinks away when it is deprived of the hormone, testosterone. Testosterone can be reduced by removing the testicles or giving shots that lower the body's testosterone levels.

LHRH Agonists—Drugs given by intramuscular injection (Lupron, Zoladex) that lower the body's testosterone level and generally cause prostate cancer to go into remission.

Margins—The edges of a prostate that have been removed. A pathologist examines these areas closely to be certain that all of the cancer was removed.

Metastatic disease—The condition in which cancer has spread beyond the organ from which it originated. When prostate cancer is found in an organ other than the prostate, it is termed a "metastasis."

Oncologist—A doctor who specializes in the medical treatment of cancers. An oncologist can be involved in the non-surgical treatment of advanced prostate cancer.

Orchiectomies—The surgical removal of the testicles. This is done to reduce blood testosterone levels and put the prostate cancer in remission.

Palliation—Refers to efforts to control the tumor and the symptoms it may produce. Palliation does not mean "cure." Generally, the term is used with patients who have advanced cancer.

Pathologist—A doctor who specializes in the diagnosis of disease by the examination of human tissue that has been removed. These tissues are examined visually and often examined under a microscope.

Percent Free–PSA—A blood test that measures how much PSA is free versus how much is bound to other blood proteins. This may help determine if cancer is present in situations when the regular PSA test is borderline high or rising.

Prostate Specific Antigen—A blood test of an enzyme made almost exclusively by the prostate. The test can be used to screen for prostate cancer. It is especially useful to monitor the results of treatment.

Radiation oncologist—A doctor who specializes in the treatment of cancer using radiation to kill the tumor cells.

Radical prostatectomy—The surgical removal of the entire prostate gland and paired seminal vesicles.

Remission—Condition in which the tumor may become invisible, dormant, inactive. Often symptoms may disappear. This can occur commonly in patients who choose hormonal deprivation for advanced cancer. Remissions do not mean "cure." The cancer will probably grow and cause symptoms again later.

Seminal vesicles—Paired organs at the bladder base that empty seminal fluid into the ejaculatory duct when a man reaches his climax. They are usually removed during a radical prostatectomy.

Stage—Describes whether the cancer is locally confined to the prostate or has spread beyond the capsule of the prostate to lymph nodes, bones, liver, lung, or other organs.

Urologist—A doctor who specializes in diseases of the urinary system, particularly those of the kidney, bladder, prostate, and testicles.

Patient Checklist

Important questions to ask your doctor that will help you choose a course of action.

➤ What is the serum PSA level (prostate specific antigen blood test)?

➤ Are you confident in the biopsy diagnosis of prostate cancer? Was there any hesitation by the pathologist to call it cancer? (If so, consider getting the microscope slides reviewed by a second pathologist.)

➤ Regarding the prostate biopsy:
  ➤ What is the Gleason grade and score?
  ➤ How many samples (tissue cores) showed cancer present?

➤ What is the stage of my disease? Has it spread?

➤ Do we want to treat this disease at all, or simply watch it?

➤ If we treat it, what is the treatment that can offer a cure?

➤ Is the disease beyond cure?

➤ How can I prepare mentally, emotionally and spiritually for treatment and healing?

Questions
You Want to Ask the Doctor Throughout Your Treatment

Comments

Your Doctor Makes to You Throughout Treatment

Diagnostic Record

DATE	TYPE OF TEST	RESULT

About the Authors

Roger E. Schultz, M.D., FACS

Roger E. Schultz, M.D., FACS, is a urologist in private practice with Urology of Virginia, P.C. in Williamsburg, Virginia. He is a native of New Jersey and a graduate of Tulane University. He received his medical degree from Mount Sinai School of Medicine in New York and completed his residency at the Hospital of the University of Pennsylvania in Philadelphia. Before entering private practice, he served as staff urologist at the Naval Hospital in Portsmouth, Virginia.

Dr. Schultz has been in private practice for fifteen years. He is a Fellow of the American College of Surgeons and former President of the Tidewater and Virginia Urological Societies. He recently served as Chief of Staff at Williamsburg Community Hospital. He lives in Williamsburg with his wife Beth Scharlop, M.D., and their two children, Alison and Sam.

A native of Virginia, Alex W. Oliver received his AB Degree in English and Journalism from Elon College. He was awarded a Ford Foundation Fellowship to study humanities at the University of Virginia early in his career as a teacher. Mr. Oliver is also a graduate of the University of Delaware with an advanced degree in Organization Management.

He is currently a professional in managing non-profit organizations. His responsibilities include lobbying, public relations and marketing, and program development on regional, state, and national levels. He is married to Libbey H. Oliver, a nationally recognized and honored expert in floral design. Recently, Governor James Gilmore appointed both of them to serve on the state's Citizens Advisory Committee to Restore the Governor's Mansion in Richmond. They reside in Williamsburg.